YOUR KNOWLEDGE HAS VALUE

AF140854

- We will publish your bachelor's and master's thesis, essays and papers

- Your own eBook and book - sold worldwide in all relevant shops

- Earn money with each sale

Upload your text at www.GRIN.com and publish for free

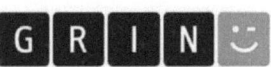

Imprint:

Copyright © 2018 GRIN Verlag, Open Publishing GmbH
Print and binding: Books on Demand GmbH, Norderstedt Germany
ISBN: 9783668623637

This book at GRIN:

https://www.grin.com/document/388326

Patrick Kimuyu

Crystal-Induced Arthropathies. Gout and Pseudogout

GRIN Publishing

GRIN - Your knowledge has value

Since its foundation in 1998, GRIN has specialized in publishing academic texts by students, college teachers and other academics as e-book and printed book. The website www.grin.com is an ideal platform for presenting term papers, final papers, scientific essays, dissertations and specialist books.

Visit us on the internet:

http://www.grin.com/

http://www.facebook.com/grincom

http://www.twitter.com/grin_com

Crystal-Induced Arthropathies: Gout and Pseudogout

Name: Patrick Kimuyu

Content

Introduction

Gout and pseudogout are believed to the most prevalent crystal-induced arthropathies in humans. These disorders occur due to the deposition of crystals in the joints and soft tissues. This results into periarticular and articular inflammation and injury. Some of the most common crystals that are responsible for arthropathies such as gout and pseudogout include hydroxyapatite, monosodium urate (MSU), calcium oxalate and calcium pyrophosphate dehydrate (CPPD) (Rothschild, 2014). In practice, gout and pseudogout are relatively different despite the fact that they are crystal-induced arthropathies, and their difference can be explained by their definitions. Gout is defined as a crystal deposition disease that is characterized by the precipitation and super-saturation of monosodium urate (MSU) in tissues. This deposition of monosodium urate crystals causes inflammation of the joints and soft tissues, and this is attributable to tissue damage. Therefore, gout is characterized by sub-acute or acute attacks of joints or the inflammation of soft tissues resulting from the deposition of monosodium urate. The clinical course of gout involves an underlying metabolic aberrancy referred to as hyperuricemia which is defined as the serum urate level of more than 6.8 mg/dL (Al-Ashkar, 2010). On the other hand, pseudogout is defined as a clinical syndrome that resembles gout, and it is caused by the deposition of calcium pyrophosphate dehydrate crystals in soft tissues and joints, resulting into the inflammation and cartilage tissue damage. Therefore, the term pseudogout emanates from the nature of its clinical presentation in which acute attacks of the joints resembles those observed in gout (Al-Ashkar, 2010). However, it is worth noting that, in pseudogout, chondrocalcinosis is the most distinctive feature for the syndrome although some patients with chondrocalcinosis do not present with pseudogout.

Epidemiology of Gout and Pseudogout

From an epidemiological perspective, gout appears to exhibit a worldwide distribution, though its prevalence rates vary significantly from one geographical location to another. In addition, its epidemiological trends exhibit demographic features, especially regarding sex, age and race. These variations are attributable to dietary, environmental and genetic influences on different global populations.

International statistics indicates that the United Kingdom records an incidence rate of 2.68 per 1000 persons. In this population, incidence rates exhibit sex related demographics in which women have a reduced incidence rate of 1.32 compared to men with 4.42. In Italy, the prevalence rate of gout is reported to be four times higher in men than in women, in which it was found to be 9.1 per 1000 populations, in 2009. This was a significant increase in the prevalence rate of gout from 6.7 per 1000 persons in 2005 (Rothschild, 2014).

In the United States, the prevalence of gout has been increasing, and this is attributable to the increase of the old population. This is evidenced by epidemiological survey data that indicate an increase in incidence rates. For instance, the incidence rate of gout is reported to have increased by 40% from 1990 to 1999 (Terkeltaub, 2008). On the other hand, the population of adults with self-reported gout increased to 3 million, in 2008 from 2.1 million people recorded in 1995. It is reported that, gout accounted for about 0.2 percent of all emergency department visits in 2008 (Garg et al. 2013). This corresponded to a prevalence rate of approximately 3.9%, primarily in adults (Rothschild, 2014).

On the other hand, sex, age and race related demographics exhibit variations. It is reported that, gout exhibits male predominance in which the global prevalence rate of gout in men is estimated to be 5.9% compared to a prevalence rate of 2% in women (Zhu, Pandya &

3

Choi, 2011). This variation in the prevalence rates of gout between men and women is attributable to the age at onset in which estrogenic hormones exert uricosuric effects. Ordinarily, uric acid levels reach the peak within the fourth and sixth decades of age, whereas women experience a uric acid level increase within the sixth and eighth decades. Therefore, it is apparent that the peak age of onset determines the prevalence rates of gout among women and men. However, it is worth noting that, lifestyle risk factors and genetic predisposition have significant influences on the prevalence of gout (Fravel & Ernst, 2011). It is also worth noting that, gout occurs more in African American populations than in whites. However, there are no epidemiological connections between blacks in the US and Africa because; gout is rare in Africa (Merriman, 2011).

In contrast to gout, epidemiological trends of pseudogout are relatively different because its prevalence exhibit age demographics, only. Clinical studies indicate that the prevalence of pseudogout occurs at a rate of 15% in populations aged between 65 and 75 years, whereas populations aged beyond 84 years record an increased prevalence rate of 40% (Al-Ashkar, 2010).

Pathophysiology

The physiology of gout is explained by the metabolic processes involved in the formation of monosodium urate crystals and their consequences in the joints and soft tissues. This is why gout is considered as a metabolic disorder because it is caused by the accumulation of uric acid precipitates in blood and tissues. Ordinarily, urate crystals are formed after the super-saturation of tissues with uric acid, a condition referred to as hyperuricemia, resulting into the precipitation of urate salts. In gout disease, monosodium urate (MSU) accumulate in the joints; thus, forming crystals under the acidic conditions and low temperatures observed in the peripheral joints. These

4

crystals are relatively insoluble under such conditions, and this leads to the accumulation of urate crystals in the affected joints as it is the case in the big toe's metatarsophalangeal joints. Ordinarily, uric acid precipitates at PH 7.4 in body fluids (Al-Ashkar, 2010). This is why high acidic conditions in the synovial fluid favor the precipitation of uric acid into urate. Polarizing microscopy shows the needlelike crystals that are formed after the precipitation of urate as light-retarding, a characteristic feature of urate crystals (Rothschild, 2014).

In theory, the pathogenic effect of the monosodium urate crystals in the soft tissue and the joints accounts for the inflammatory crystal arthropathy that is observed in the gout disease. In the body, uric acid is formed from the metabolism of purine nucleotides in which inosine and hypoxanthine are formed as the precursors of uric acid. In purine metabolism, hypoxanthine is broken down to xanthine which is, in turn metabolized to uric acid. Ordinarily, uric acid is formed from the subsequent oxidation of hypoxanthine to xanthine, and then from xanthine to uric acid under the catalytic influence of the xanthine oxidase enzyme (Al-Ashkar, 2010). Therefore, uric acid is the final product of purine metabolism in the body.

In gout disease, physiologic conditions in the affected tissues and fluids, especially the synovial fluid cause the conversion of uric acid to urate which is not required in the human body. It has been found out that there is no biological pathway for the degradation of urate as it is the case in other animals such as reptiles and birds. Therefore, its elimination from the body is relatively difficult, although minimal amounts are eliminated through the intestinal and urinary tracts. It is believed that the inability of the human body to eliminate large amounts of urate leads to hyperuricemia. As a result, urate saturates the synovial fluid in the joints and soft tissues where it precipitates to form crystals which are responsible for the development of tophi and tissue damage. These changes in the constituents of the synovial fluid, especially the presence of urate deposits trigger an immune response in which macrophages and monocytes are mobilized to clears the urate crystals through phagocytosis. As a result, pro-inflammatory chemicals such as chemokines and cytokines are released into the surrounding tissues, and this triggers an influx of neutrophils into the synovial cavity. In addition, the release of these chemicals triggers acute inflammatory reaction cascade, and this explains why inflammation occurs in the affected tissues. However, biochemical studies indicate that there is a self-limited inflammatory process in which cell-mediated anti-inflammatory process is initiated to counter inflammation in the affected tissues, although the mechanism for this process is not well understood. Therefore, it is believed that the self-limited inflammatory process explains why the pathological course of gout resolves spontaneously on average of one to two weeks (Al-Ashkar, 2010).

Another mechanism that explains the pathophysiology of both gout and pseudogout is the role of interleukin 1 (IL-1) and inflammasome. This mechanism is involved in the inflammation induced by calcium pyrophosphate dehydrate (CPPD) in pseudogout and monosodium urate (MSU) in gout. In this mechanism, cryopyrin inflammasome triggers an inflammatory cascade that involves the activation of interleukin-1 after it detects urate crystals, primarily monosodium urate and calcium pyrophosphate dehydrate (CPPD) (Choi et al. 2004). As a result, inflammation occurs in the affected areas.

In general, it is believed that the presence of urate crystals; monosodium urate and calcium pyrophosphate dehydrate, in the synovial tissues and soft tissues serves as a prerequisite the gout disease. However, it is worth noting that the presence of urate crystals on the cartilage surface and the synovial fluid do not necessary mean that joint inflammation occurs. In reality, a gout attack is usually triggered by two principal factors. In most cases, a gout attack is triggered by the release of crystals into the synovial tissues owing to the partial dissolution of microtophi

6

that are caused by changes in the serum urate levels. The second factor that triggers a gout attack is the precipitation of urate crystals, especially in a supersaturated microenvironment. This is attributable to the release of urate from cellular damage. In these two mechanisms, urate crystals interact with the receptors of macrophages and dendritic cells, and trigger a danger signal; thus, activating the innate immune response which results into an inflammation of the affected tissue (Liu-Bryan et al., 2005). As a result, interleukin- 1β is released into the surrounding tissues (Akahoshi, Murakami & Kitasato, 2007). It is believed that interleukin- 1β triggers the release of pro-inflammatory cytokines including the tumor necrosis factor (TNF-α), interleukin-6, interleukin-8 and neutrophil chemotactic factors (Martinon, 2010). In addition, neutrophil phagocytosis triggers further production of inflammatory mediator; thus, resulting into advanced inflammation of the synovial tissues (Rothschild, 2014).

Moreover, recent studies indicate that genetic factors play a significant role in the pathophysiology of gout and pseudogout. This phenomenon has been studied through genome-wide associated studies in which some genetic variants have been found to modulate uric acid levels. In these studies, genetic variants of ABCG2 were reported to have physiological connections with high levels of serum uric acid concentrations in which its effects were found to be stronger in men than women. On the other hand, genetic variants of SLC2A9/GLUT9 have been found to lower the levels of uric acid in women more than men. Therefore, GLUT9 and ABCG2 influence the transportation of urate, and these variants explain the pathogenesis of gout (Choi, Zhu & Mount, 2010).

Clinical Presentation

Clinical presentation of gout exhibits an array of signs and symptoms. Ordinarily, gout affects the lower extremity joints such as the metatarsophalangeal joints. It also occurs in the knees, ankles, wrists, feet and elbow joints. Moreover, acute gout has been observed to occur in the bursae including prepatellar and olecranon bursae in which it causes bursitis (Al-Ashkar, 2010).

Regarding the onset, gout attacks are believed to begin abruptly in which they reach maximum intensity in 8-12 hours. In the case of pseudogout, the onset of an attack resembles that of acute gout. However, it is worth noting that an insidious onset that occurs for several days suggests the presence of pseudogout. In most cases, untreated gout results into intensive polyarticular attacks, especially in the upper extremity and proximal joints. These attacks have been observed to last longer than the initial attacks witnessed at the onset of gout, and they occur more often (Rothschild, 2014).

In most cases, inflammation of the synovial tissues is considered as the principal sign of gout. Other signs observed in physical findings are tenderness of the affected tissues and erythema. However, it is worth noting that, erythema associated with gout may resemble cellulitis in some cases; thus, caution must be observed during the diagnosis of gout. Another sign for gout is the presence of conjunctival nodules in the eyes of the affected patient that contain crystals. In addition, tophi in the soft tissues, especially in the toes, the helix of the ear, prepatellar bursa and fingers are suggestive of gout or pseudogout (Rothschild, 2014).

On the other hand, gout presents in different symptoms. In practice, fever, blurred vision and band keratopathy are considered as the most significant symptoms of gout. In addition, gout is presented by migratory polyarthritis and anterior uveitis, although these characteristics are rare

8

(Rothschild, 2014). Moreover, gout is manifested by leukocytosis, malaise and the elevation of acute phase reactants.

Complications of gout are manifested by several signs and symptoms. Some of the most common clinical characteristics include severe degenerative arthritis, urate nephropathy and spinal cord impingement. Other clinical characteristics are renal stones and fractures in joints, especially in patients with tophaceous gout (Martinon & Glimcher, 2006).

In pseudogout, clinical manifestations range from asymptomatic to gout-like features. In some circumstances, pseudogout is manifested by rheumatoid arthritis-like or pseudo-osteoarthritis conditions. It is worth noting that, it is relatively difficult to distinguish gout from pseudogout by the use of their clinical manifestations because pseudogout mimics gout. Therefore, the most reliable distinction is based on the synovial fluid analysis (Al-Ashkar, 2010).

Diagnosis and Differential Diagnosis of Gout and Pseudogout

Diagnosis

In practice, synovial fluid analysis is considered as the gold standard in the diagnosis of gout and pseudogout. Therefore, synovial aspiration is recommended for microscopic analysis. It is believed that the analysis of synovial fluid is the most appropriate diagnostic approach for the diagnosis of gout and pseudogout because it allows for the gross examination of the synovial fluid for color and turbidity. For instance, physical examination of the synovial fluid enables the determination of inflammation conditions in gout or pseudogout. Ordinarily, turbid or purulent appearance of the synovial fluid in the syringe is suggestive of an inflammatory condition which is a characteristic of gout and pseudogout. On the other hand, a transparent appearance of the synovial fluid is suggestive of non-inflammatory condition, and this can be used to rule out the absence of these diseases. However, it is worth noting that gross appearance of the synovial fluid is not considered as an adequate diagnostic; thus, diagnosis must be confirmed through the use of polarized microscopic examination. In addition, gram staining and culture procedures are performed, in order to confirm the diagnosis. In microscopic examination, the presence of leukocytosis in the synovial fluid sample indicates inflammation, whereas the white blood cell count is used to evaluate the degree of inflammation (Al-Ashkar, 2010).

On the other hand, crystal analysis with polarized a microscope helps in the detection and identification of urate crystals in the synovial fluid. Ordinarily, monosodium urate crystals are distinguished from calcium pyrophosphate through the use of birefringence, shape and color. Monosodium urate crystals exhibit a stronger birefringence than CPPD. Another distinctive characteristic between MSU and CPPD is the shape of the crystals. MSU crystals appear needle-like with sharp edges, whereas CPPD appears rod-like in shape. Moreover, urate crystals exhibit color variations under polarized light in which MSU appear yellow in color parallel to the polarizer compared to the blue color of CPPD crystals (Al-Ashkar, 2010).

Radiography plays a principal role in identifying chondrocalcinosis which is a characteristic of pseudogout. Therefore, radiographs are used for determining the extent of joint degeneration and the confirmation of clinical impression. However, it is worth noting that radiography is not required for the diagnosis of pseudogout where CPPD crystals are revealed in polarized microscopic examination (Al-Ashkar, 2010). As such, primary diagnosis is adequate for the diagnosis of pseudogout. In practice, primary diagnosis, analysis of the synovial fluid, is considered for gout and pseudogout diagnosis over radiography because; the latter does not show the urate crystal characteristics.

In addition, blood tests such as the evaluation of urate levels and creatinine in the patient's blood circulation are useful in the identification of other co-morbid diseases. They are also useful in monitoring drug toxicity during the management of gout or pseudogout. In most cases, blood tests reveal hyperuricemia in the blood circulation. However, it is worth noting that hyperuricemia is not considered as a significant clinical manifestation of gout because; this condition can also be caused by diet and some drugs such as diuretics used for other conditions (Rothschild, 2014). Therefore, blood tests are used in determining hypouricemic therapy, especially in chronic gout, but not for diagnosis purposes.

The other diagnosis used in gout and pseudogout is the urine test. A 24-hour uric acid evaluation helps in determining uric acid levels in urine. This approach is useful during the management of gout in which the levels of urate are used in choosing the most appropriate therapy, especially when uricosuric agents are used. Ordinarily, urine tests are not used for the diagnosis of gout because they can be influenced by genetic and dietary factors.

Differential Diagnosis

Differential diagnosis for gout and pseudogout include rheumatoid arthritis, osteoarthritis and septic arthritis. In most cases, gout presents as rheumatoid arthritis (Montgomery, 2008). Therefore, it is worth carrying out differential diagnosis to differentiate between gout and rheumatoid arthritis. In comparison, both conditions affect the synovial fluid of the joints. In gout, pain in the joints is experienced at the time of gout attack, whereas rheumatoid arthritis is characterized by joint stiffness and pain after long rest, especially in the morning. In diagnosis, radiography is useful in differentiating gout from rheumatoid arthritis. This is so because; radiography enables the detection of erosions involved in the arthropathy. Ordinarily, well-defined erosions with overhanging edges and sclerotic margins are usually a characteristic feature in gout. Therefore, the absence of periarticular osteopenia and joint space narrowing are suggestive of rheumatoid arthritis (Choi, MacKenzie & Dalinka, 2006).

Septic arthritis is the second condition that resembles gout. This condition is caused by bacterial infection in which joint inflammation occurs in the large joints such as the hip and knee. In both gout and septic arthritis inflammation in the joints is observed (Hayes, Hoyt & Peard, 2007). Therefore, diagnosis involves gram staining, white blood cell count and culture. Ordinarily, growth in synovial fluid cultures helps in differentiating septic arthritis from gout.

Moreover, osteoarthritis is used in the differential diagnosis for gout and pseudogout. This condition presents as localized joint pains, but it does not manifest inflammation as it is the case in gout and pseudogout. In general, osteoarthritis is not characterized by systemic symptoms (Grogan & Sovani, 2013). In practice, these conditions are differentiated through the use of microscopy and radiography in which the absence of urate deposits in the synovial fluid suggests osteoarthritis. On the other hand, radiography for osteoarthritis reveals irregular tear and wear of the bone joints, whereas gout shows well-defined erosions with overhanging edges and sclerotic margins.

Diagnostics for Gout and Pseudogout

In the diagnosis for gout, synovial fluid analysis are ordered including, gram staining, culture and microscopic examination. Gram staining enables healthcare professionals in the gout diagnosis through carrying out laboratory procedures that determine the presence of infections by bacteria. This is significant in the diagnosis of gout because; inflammations in the joints can be caused by bacterial and fungal infections. It is also useful in the diagnosis of pseudogout because it helps in determining co-morbid conditions in patients. On the other hand, microbial cultures help in determining the presence of pathogens in the synovial fluids. In practice, the absence of microbial growth in cultures of synovial fluid samples obtained in inflamed joints combined with microscopy is indicative of gout.

Treatment/Management

In practice, the treatment of gout and pseudogout depends primarily on the clinical presentation of the disease. However, treatment focuses on addressing acute attacks and the prevention of future attacks, as well as, preventing the development of gouty arthropathy. In general, the treatment of gout involves three principal stages; the treatment of an acute gout attacks, prevention of acute flares through the use of prophylaxis and decreasing urate levels in the body of gout patients.

In asymptomatic hyperuricemia, hypouricemic agents are used to lower urate levels, and this leads to the elimination of the associated symptoms. However, asymptomatic hyperuricemia does not require treatment. Instead, treatment of the underlying co-morbid conditions is recommended in alleviating their conditions (Reginato et al., 2012).

On the other hand, acute attacks caused by acute intermittent gout are managed with anti-inflammatory drugs including corticosteroids, NSAIDs and nonsteroidal agents. However, colchicine has always been used as the primary drug in the treatment of gout. Ideally, the choice of the agents used in the treatment of acute gout depends on the patient's tolerance. In most cases, patients manifest tolerance to a given drug, whereas others are intolerant. Therefore, it is worth determining the toxicity of these drugs after the initial therapy. In cases where patients prove intolerant to a given drug, supplementation is recommended to prevent adverse treatment outcomes (Rothschild, 2014).

In chronic tophaceous gout, the focus of treatment approaches is to reduce the precipitation of uric acid through lowering urate levels. In practice, the therapeutic target for the management of chronic tophaceous gout is set at less than 6 mg/dL. Some of the agents used in the management of chronic tophaceous gout include allopurinol and uricosuric drugs such as sulfinpyrazone and probenecid (Al-Ashkar, 2010). These agents inhibit the key enzymes involved in the purine metabolism such as xanthine oxidase which catalyses the conversion of xanthine to uric acid. For instance, allopurinol acts as an inhibitor of this enzyme; therefore, it prevents the production of uric acid in the patient's body (Borstad et al., 2004).

Conclusion

In a brief conclusion, gout and pseudogout are metabolic disorders that are caused by crystal deposition in the synovial and soft tissues in the joints. These diseases account for the highest percentage of crystal arthropathies. Ordinarily, gout is caused by the deposition of monosodium urate in the joints; whereas pseudogout is caused by the deposition of calcium pyrophosphate dehydrate. Pseudogout mimics the clinical manifestations of gout and other co-morbid conditions such as rheumatoid arthritis and osteoarthritis. However, these diseases manifest diverse epidemiological trends in which gout exhibits sex, race and age related demographics. Despite the lack of extensive research on pseudogout, demographic features have not been identified; thus, the prevalence ratio is 50:50 between men and women, although these trends are influenced by diet and environmental factors (Lee, Terkeltaub & Kavanaugh, 2006).

Diagnosis for these conditions involves the analysis of the synovial fluid, blood tests, radiography, and urine tests. On the other hand, treatment focuses on the elimination of the symptoms and the prevention of acute attacks.

References

Akahoshi ,T., Murakami ,Y., & Kitasato, H. (2007). Recent Advances in Crystal-Induced Acute
Inflammation. *Curr Opin Rheumatol.*, 19(2):146-50.

Al-Ashkar, F. (2010). *Gout and Pseudogout.* Retrieved from
http://www.clevelandclinicmeded.com/medicalpubs/diseasemanagement/rheumatology/g
out-and-pseudogout/

Borstad, G. C. et al. (2004). Colchicine for Prophylaxis of Acute Flares When Initiating
Allopurinol for Chronic Gouty Arthritis. *J Rheumatol.*, 31: 2429-2432.

Choi, H. K. et al. (2004). Alcohol Intake and Risk of Incident Gout in Men: A Prospective Study.
Lancet, 363: 1277-1281.

Choi, M. H., MacKenzie, J. D. & Dalinka, M. K. (2006). Imaging Features of Crystal-Induced
Arthropathy. *Rheum Dis Clin North Am.*, 32: 427-446.

Choi, H., Zhu, Y. & Mount, D. B. (2010). Genetics of Gout. *Curr Opin Rheumatol.*, 22(2):144-
51.

Fravel, M. A. & Ernst, M. E. (2011). Management of Gout in the Older Adult. *Am J Geriatr
Pharmacother*, 9(5):271-85.

Garg, R. et al. (2013). Gout-Related Health Care Utilization in US Emergency Departments,
2006 through 2008. *Arthritis Care Res (Hoboken),* 65(4):571-7.

Grogan, S. & Sovani, S. (2013). Osteoarthritis Detection, Pathophysiology, and Current/Future
Treatment Strategies. *Orthopaedic Nursing*, 32(1): 25-36.

Hayes, K., Hoyt, S. & Peard, A. S. (2007). Differential Diagnosis of a Patient Presenting With a
Knee Effusion. *Advanced Emergency Nursing Journal*, 29(3): 209-227.

Lee, S. J., Terkeltaub, R. A. & Kavanaugh, A. (2006). Recent Developments in Diet And Gout. *Curr Opin Rheumatol.*, 18: 193-198.

Liu-Bryan, R. et al. (2005). Innate Immunity Conferred By Toll-Like Receptors 2 And 4 And Myeloid Differentiation Factor 88 Expression Is Pivotal To Monosodium Urate Monohydrate Crystal-Induced Inflammation. *Arthritis Rheum.*, 52(9):2936-46.

Martinon, F. & Glimcher, L. H. (2006). Gout: New Insights into an Old Disease. *J Clin Invest.*, 116(8):2073-5.

Martinon, F. (2010). Mechanisms of Uric Acid Crystal-Mediated Autoinflammation. *Immunol Rev.*, 233(1):218-32.

Merriman, T. R. (2011). Population Heterogeneity in the Genetic Control of Serum Urate. *Semin Nephrol.*, 31(5):420-5.

Montgomery, M. (2008). Gout: Tips on diagnosis, treatment, and patient education. *The Nurse Practitioner: The American Journal of Primary Health Care*, 33(12): 28-32.

Reginato, A. M. et al. (2012). The Genetics of Hyperuricaemia and Gout. *Nat Rev Rheumatol.*, 8(10):610-21.

Rothschild, B. M. (2014). *Gout and Pseudogout.* Retrieved from http://emedicine.medscape.com/article/329958-overview#showall

Terkeltaub, R. A. (2008). Gout: Recent advances and emerging therapies. *Rheumatic Disease Clinics Update*, 3(1):1-9.

Zhu, Y., Pandya, B. J. & Choi, H. K. (2011). Prevalence of Gout And Hyperuricemia in The US General Population: The National Health and Nutrition Examination Survey 2007-2008. *Arthritis Rheum.*, 63(10):3136-41.

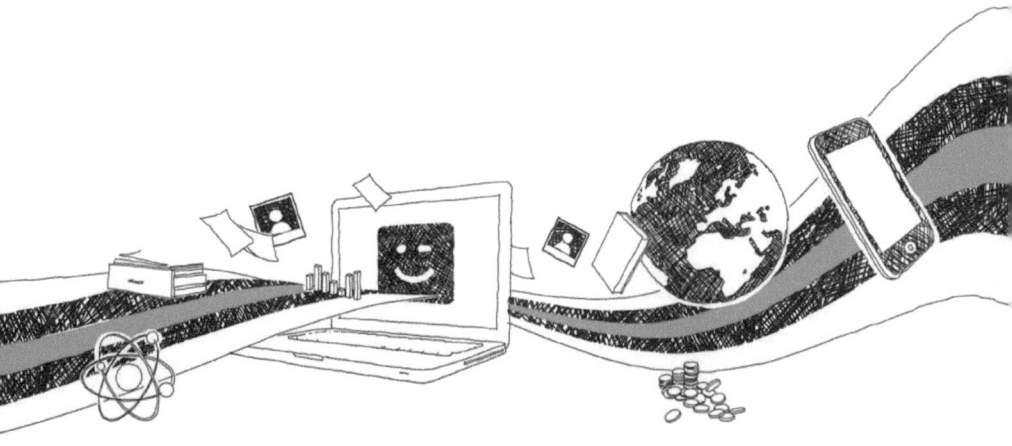
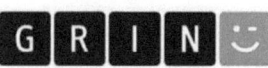